Plant Based Diet for Beginners

Your Starting-Point Guide to Great Food, Good
Health and Natural Weight Loss;
With 30 Proven, Simple and Tasty Recipes

AUTHOR: REBECCA BELLIS

Legal & Disclaimer

The information contained in this book and its contents is not designed to replace or take the place of any form of medical or professional advice; and is not meant to replace the need for independent medical, financial, legal or other professional advice or services, as may be required. The content and information in this book have been provided for educational and entertainment purposes only.

The content and information contained in this book have been compiled from sources deemed reliable, and it is accurate to the best of the Author's knowledge, information, and belief. However, the Author cannot guarantee its accuracy and validity and cannot be held liable for any errors and omissions. Further, changes are periodically made to this book as and when needed. Where appropriate and necessary, you must consult a professional (including but not limited to your doctor, attorney, financial advisor or such other professional advisor) before using any of the suggested remedies, techniques, or information in this book.

Upon using the contents and information contained in this book, you agree to hold harmless the Author from and against any damages, costs, and expenses, including any legal fees potentially resulting from the application of any of the information provided by this book. This disclaimer applies to any loss, damages or injury caused by the use and application, whether directly or indirectly, of any advice or information

Table of Content

INTRODUCTION

This book reveals to you how easy it is to change your life and reap all the benefits a plant based diet has to offer!

The Plant based diet is a low fat, high carb and protein diet that has similar qualities like Vegan, Vegetarian, Mediterranean, China study, and raw food diets.

Coming to facts, there are many exceptional gains of advantages of the Plant based diet plan, but a lot of people missing secure manner to fat loss forever with full energy to hold healthy life for a long time.

Following a Plant based diet comes with essential benefits:

- Lose Weight: weight loss occurs with the increased consumption of fiber and vitamins, which is an effect of switching to a plant-based diet

- Reduced Risk of Chronic Diseases: Plant based diets work as a medicine to reduce the number of doctor visits

- More Energy: Whole food Plant based diet is high in vitamins, minerals, antioxidants, and many other nutrients

- Less Expensive: beans and legumes are great sources of protein that cost significantly less than an equivalent amount of meat

- Better Digestion: fruits and vegetables are high in fiber that is an essential nutrient for healthy digestion

Additionally, you will get tips and tricks to ensure that your dietary mini habits will develop as quickly as possible, including how to totally commit to the new food regimen.

After that, you will discover 30 best plant-based recipes which will help you to get and keep a lean body without losing energy and vitality levels!

CHAPTER 1:
What is the Plant Based Diet and Why it Works

The plant based diet is low-fat, high carb and protein diet that has similar qualities like vegan, Mediterranean, and raw food diets.

Why plant-based diet: Plant-based diet allows easy absorption of nutrients straight into the bloodstream and helps to heal the body and digestive system very fast and aids in weight control but meat items will slow down the digestive system.

Protein myth: Plants contain 30 to 40 percent of greens are a great source of protein in the body, which provide protein in the form of amino acids and building blocks of protein. This makes the body to utilize them easier than other animal products and easier for the digestive system. If you feel that you required additional protein for your body due to heavy workouts, feel free to add plant based protein powder in your food or juices or smoothies, while making yummy and delicious plant based recipes (some of the plant-based protein powder are pea protein powder, hemp protein powder, soy protein powder, brown rice protein powder, pumpkin protein powder).

Eating vegetables and natural products as a significant aspect of our day to day life will help to overcome some genuine medical issues. Most fruits and vegetables are normally low in fat and calories, but fruits have low fat and more fiber and water, this makes digestive system healthy because fruits have low sodium-content with natural sugar.

Fruits and vegetables will have some similar nutrients, micronutrients are a class of supplements that incorporate vitamins, minerals, and phytonutrients that are essential for the body to maintain the proper healthy functioning of the organs.

Leafy vegetables have more micronutrients than any other vegetables or fruits like iron, calcium, and magnesium. This plays a key role in the proper functioning of the nervous system as well as the immune system.

Root vegetables are the powerhouses of minerals, vitamins and also additionally supply carbohydrates, especially complex-carbohydrates, which gradually supply constant energy to the body.

If you feel that you required additional protein for your body due to heavy workouts, feel free to add plant based protein powder in your food or juices or smoothies (some of the plant based protein powder are pea protein powder, hemp protein powder, soy protein powder, brown rice protein powder, pumpkin protein powder).

CHAPTER 2: Benefits of Plant Based Diet

When you start eating plant based food, automatically body starts losing weight immediately, and you will feel and look better from the inside out. Some of the health benefits you will achieve while eating include:

Weight loss: After trying plant based recipes, you will be surprised to learn that this recipe is one of the best ways to get lean body without any difficulty because this recipe contains high quantity of water filled with green leafy veggies with high fiber content, which helps you stay full for a long time and also reduce cravings for junk food.

Rich nutrient: In case of plant based food all ingredients are fully loaded with vitamins, minerals, antioxidants, water, fiber, phytonutrients, anti-inflammatory substances, and chlorophyll. This chlorophyll has a similar structure to hemoglobin in blood, which acts as cleansing blood transfusion.

Easy to digest: The plant-based foods contain more valuable nutrients than any other food items like meat and take less time to digest. These foods contain high quantity of phytonutrients, which keeps your digestive system functioning properly and improves health by reducing future diseases.

Detoxification: Normally our body tries to eliminate toxins, but due to lack of organic food, it will slow down the body's detoxification system and causes weight gain; we have to take plant based foods because it will produce fiber, which helps you in cleansing your digestive system and eliminate toxins.

Hydration: Normally, staying hydrated gives energy and helps your brain, immune system and digestive system work properly without any defects. An easy way to check yourself whether you are hydrated or dehydrated by looking at your urine color. If it is intense yellow color, then you are dehydrated, and that means our body is directly saying that we forgot to drink sufficient water due to our busy work.

Blood sugar improvement: Blood sugar levels will be improved because it reduces glucose and glycated hemoglobin in the body.

Blood pressure lowering: Researchers identified that diet will lead to lower the blood pressure and helps to reduce strokes and heart diseases.

Cholesterol Problems: Helps to reduce the bad cholesterol and increases good cholesterol, which is necessary for the body.

Acne: Recent human studies have shown a drastic drop in acne lesions and skin inflammation over 10-12 weeks.

Energy: This gives you more reliable power which keeps your body more energized during a day

Anti-aging: When you start eating plant-based food, you can see changes not only inside but also outside of the body, especially after toxin free. Slowly it will start eliminating wrinkles, acne and dark circles under eye and makes your face young again.

CHAPTER 3:
Protein Source

When you start and include plant-based diet in your life, most of the people could have misconceptions concerning protein deficiency because protein will play an essential role to build and maintain proper tissues for a lean body but we can get the right amount of protein for our body by consuming plant-based food products also.

Protein requirements: Recent research shows that vegetarians and vegan food regimen humans are exceeding their protein requirements; recommended protein for a healthy body is 0.5 grams per pound of body weight. For example: in case your weight is a 60 lb, you can multiply 60 x 0.5 = 30 grams of protein for the perfect healthy lean body.

Great Source of Protein

We have established that amino acids play a crucial role in constructing protein blocks in our body due to the fact the body can't produce by means of itself. There are 22 varieties of amino acids, among them nine are vital. Let's see details of 9 vital amino acids, its duties and from which plants we can get them.

Leucine: Leucine is for stimulating muscles and which plays an important role in strengthening muscle growth and manipulates your blood sugar, insulin levels, regulate depression. Some of the best-plant based food that help to get this amino acid is sesame seeds, avocados, apple, blueberries, banana, turnip greens, pumpkin, peas, watercress, fig, sunflower seeds, kidney beans, raisins, olives, and soy.

Isoleucine: Isoleucine is to provide energy and hemoglobin and additionally allows nitrogen growth in the muscles. You can get this amino acid in oats, spinach, hemp seeds, kiwis, cranberries, cabbage, almonds, cashews, beans, chia seeds, lentils, quinoa and brown rice.

Lysine: Lysine helps in calcium absorption and collagen development to strengthen bones. Due to deficiency of lysine results in fatigue, nausea, and depletion of muscle. Some of the plant-based foods items help to get this amino acid are parsley, avocados, watercress, soy, hemp seeds, spirulina, chia seeds, cashews, almonds.

Methionine with the help of sulfur it forms cartilage in the body. Deficiency of methionine in the body creates tissue damage, arthritis pain, and weak recovery/healing. Some of the plant-based foods that help to get required methionine are oats, sunflower seeds, wheat, whole grain rice, onions, cacao, legumes, beans, sunflower seed butter, Brazil nuts, hemp seeds, chia seeds, figs, and raisins.

Phenylalanine: Phenylalanine facilitates to form thyroid hormones and brain-boosting chemical compounds. Deficiency of this amino acid leads to brain fog, lack of urge for any food and energy, depression and reminiscence issues. Some of the plant -based foods that help to get required phenylalanine are leafy veggies, olives, avocado, berries, pumpkin, figs, beans, rice, peanuts, and almonds.

Threonine: Threonine is one of the critical amino acids supports your immune system, nervous system, heart, and liver. Additionally, it will provide glycine and serine to the body, which plays a vital role in the healthy growth of skin, hair, bones, and nails. Some of the plant- based foods that help to get required threonine are leafy veggies, soya beans, wheat, spirulina, watercress, sprouted grains, hemp seeds, sesame seeds and chia seeds.

Tryptophan: Tryptophan is a relaxing amino acid, acts as a neurotransmitter for happiness, stress, tidiness, and depression. Some of the plant based foods that help to get required tryptophan are oats, spinach, beets, mushrooms, celery, candy potatoes, squash, asparagus, peas, all lettuces, oranges, carrots, pepper, and onions.

Valine: Valine plays a major role in growth and repair of muscle/tissues. Some of the plant-based food that helps to get required Valine are broccoli, beans, legumes, sprouted grains, blueberries, cranberries, apricots, sesame seeds and peanuts.

Histidine: Histidine acts as brain messengers and also enables in detoxifying the red and white blood cells in the blood. Deficiency of this amino acid in the body causes sexual disorder, arthritis and improves the risk of the AIDS virus. Some of the plant-based foods that help to get required histidine are buckwheat, potatoes, cauliflower, cantaloupe, legumes, corn, rice, wheat, and rye.

CHAPTER 4:
Tips and Tricks

Depending on your next day timetable you can prepare required ingredients in advance to avoid last movement confusions and also you can make a right healthy meal based on your goal (weight loss, energy, and vitality or detox).

Basic step: Begin each day with a few glasses of water and followed by a cup of detox tea with natural sweetener which will provide cleansing support for your kidneys and liver and helps to flush away toxins from the body.

If you feel that you require additional protein for your body due to heavy workouts, feel free to add plant based protein powder in your food or juices or smoothies (some of the plant based protein powder are pea protein powder, hemp protein powder, soy protein powder, brown rice protein powder, pumpkin protein powder).

Basic Mistakes

Less protein intake: In a plant-based diet, we should understand consuming more protein will lead to gluconeogenesis, which converts the amino acids to glucose and leads to increase glucose levels in the body.

More nuts intake: Nuts are stuffed with lots of protein and fat but remember they have stuffed with lots of calories also. So, try to consume nuts in minimum quantity or replace with fruits.

More fat intake: Remember that intake of fat should be less than both protein and carbs. Sometimes people's intake of fat is almost equal to protein, but it is wrong.

The Same type of meal: When you are making the same kind of meal every time, you will be bored and lose interest in the main goal to main lean body and gain energy. So, to keep your spirit high, make and discover your own recipes.

Basic Exercises

For any diet, necessary training is the key to start a new habit, for example, 10-15 minutes of body movements per day will help a lot. Let's see some of the necessary changes that contribute to losing weight faster when you are on a diet.

Park and walk: I think you already heard about this technique, but I am 100% sure that this works. Instead of parking in front of your office or workplace, park little far for next parking lot, which makes you walk and helps you to maintain proper blood flow in your body.

Mostly prefer staircase: Instead of using the elevator in an office or any other place, use staircase which squeezes your muscles of the body and keeps you away from joints, ligaments, and bone pains. Doing this will burn more calories.

Take advantage of shopping: If you don't have a big shopping list, then this is the right time to use your body. Keep the bags on your shoulders and walk for selecting items and carrying the heavy grocery items with your hands is a great workout and the same time you will be finishing your shopping for whole weeks also.

Stretch yourself: Sitting in front of your desk or computer is extremely hard for the body, but there are lots ways that you can work while sitting. One of the best ways is toning your legs at regular intervals and whenever you go to the toilet or coffee stretch your whole body and go. Upgrade to the stability ball instead of sitting in a regular chair.

Prepare yourself: Do you know that cooking food by yourself for breakfast, lunch, and dinner is also an exercise which helps your body and tries to use more calories and avoid future health problems?

CHAPTER 5:
Brief Overview of Plant Based Food

Eating vegetables and natural products as a major aspect of our day to day life will help to overcome some genuine medical issues. Most fruits and vegetables are normally low in fat and calories. Fruits and vegetables will have some similar micronutrients - a class of supplements that incorporate vitamins, minerals, and phytonutrients that are essential for the body to maintain the proper healthy functioning of the organs.

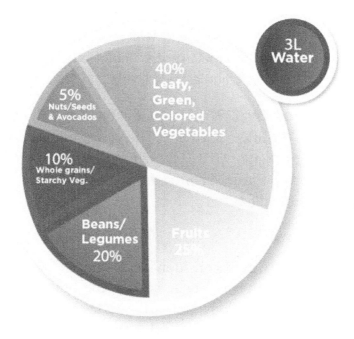

Leafy vegetables have more micronutrients than any other vegetables or fruits like iron, calcium, and magnesium. This plays a key role in the proper functioning of the nervous system as well as the immune system.

Root vegetables are the powerhouses of minerals, vitamins and also additionally supply carbohydrates, especially complex-carbohydrates, which gradually supply constant energy to the body.

Fats and Oil's

When you are on the plant based diet, fats will play a significant role in your daily calorie intake. Fats are essential to our bodies, so make sure that you consume right type of fats to avoid wrong leading. The essential fats that play a vital role in a diet are:

Polyunsaturated fats: These are usually available in the form of vegetable oils and processed polyunsaturated fats are bad for the body, which will worsen HDL/LDL cholesterol levels and natural polyunsaturated fats are good for the body to improve HDL/LDL cholesterol levels.

Monounsaturated fats: These fats are well known and used for a healthy lifestyle. These improve the insulin resistance and better HDL/LDL cholesterol levels. Olive and sunflower oil are significant examples of healthy monounsaturated fats.

Sweeteners

The vast majority of us consider "sugar" for coffee or espresso, but in subjective terms, sugar is only the building blocks of carbohydrates in the body. Research studies say that sugar and weight gain is tremendous. Sugar is the one of the main cause of every modern health problem.

- Sugar must be used by the liver and can't be utilized for vitality by your body's cells, similar effects on the liver as alcohol.

- Sugar reacts with proteins and fats in our bodies 7 times more than glucose.

- Sugar increases uric acid production in the body, which causes kidney stones.

- Abundance sugar alone can cause every one of the issues related to the metabolic disorder (heart disease, obesity, diabetes).

Staying away from sweet items is the best bet. It will help control your cravings to a minimal level, which mainly contributes to achieving success on a diet. If you like to have a sweet, best choice is an alternative sweetener:

- Liquid Stevia
- Erythritol
- Liquid Sucralose
- Xylitol
- Monk Fruit
- Coconut (palm) sugar

Plant Based Food List

Vegetables	Avocados, Bell Peppers, Eggplants, Cauliflower, Celery, Asparagus, Tomatoes, Cucumber, Onions, Cabbage, Leeks, Artichokes, Kohlrabi, Okra, Green Onions, Brussels Sprouts, Broccoli
Green Leafy Veg	Radicchio, Lettuce, Turnip Greens, Rapini, Spinach, Dandelion, Swiss Chard, Seaweeds, Arugula (Rocket), Collard Greens, Watercress, Endive, Kale, Beet Top, Mustard Greens, Chicory, Bok Choy
Root Vegetables	Sweet Potatoes, Cassava, Yams, Radish, Carrots, Rutabaga, Beets, Parsnips, Turnips, Jerusalem Artichokes
Winter Squash	Pumpkin, Butternut Squash, Acorn Squash, Spaghetti Squash
Summer Squash	Zucchini, Yellow Summer Squash, Yellow Crookneck Squash
Fruit	Coconut, Passion Fruit, Bananas, Cantaloupe, Persimmon, Apples, Pomegranates, Oranges, Cherries, Blueberry, Strawberry, Raspberry, Cranberry, Blackberry, Plantains, Lime, Grapefruit, Kiwi, Pears, Apricot, Peaches, Honeydew Melon, Nectarines, Lychee, Plums, , Pineapple, Watermelon, Papaya, Grapes, Lemon, Mango, Olives, Figs, Tangerine, Dates
Nuts & Seeds.	Pistachios, Brazil Nuts, Sunflower Seeds, Sesame Seeds, Chia Seeds, Pumpkin Seeds, Flax Seeds, Pecans, Walnuts, Chestnuts, Pine Nuts, Macadamia Nuts, Hazelnuts, Almonds, Cashews
Herbs	Tarragon, Parsley, Lavender, Coriander, Mint, Basil, Rosemary, Chives, Oregano, Dill, Bay Leaves, Thyme, Sage

Spices & Others	Horseradish, Black Pepper, Ginger, Mustard Seeds, Garlic, Onions, Cayenne Pepper, Hot Peppers, Nutmeg, Star Anise, Turmeric, Fennel Seeds, Chilies, Cloves, Cumin, Vanilla, Cinnamon, Paprika
Legumes	Black Beans, Green Soybeans, Edamame, Chickpeas, Chia Seeds, Flax Seeds, Lentils, Tempeh, Sunflower Seeds, Northen Beans, Peas, Pinto
Grains	Oats, Tortilla, Brown Rice, Barley, Pasta, Bulgar, Buckwheat, Quinoa, Millet, Whole Wheat Bread
Fats & Oils	Canola, Extra Virgin Oil, Flaxseed Oil, Avocado Oil, Olive Oil

CHAPTER 6:
Perfect 21 Day's Meal Plan

DAY	BREAKFAST	LUNCH	SNACK	DINNER
Day 1	Avocado Sesame Bread	Pure Green Soup	Pure Green Smoothie	Yummy spaghetti squash
Day 2	Blueberry Chia Oats	Lentil Green salad	Creamy Apple Cake	Hot Kimchi Bowl
Day 3	Vegetable Tortilla	Coconut Potato Flower Stew	Pure Honey Basil	Linguine with Green Sauce
Day 4	Blueberry Chia Oats	Peanut Pumpkin Soup	Brain-Boosting Smoothie	Mixed Beans Chili
Day 5	Blueberry Pancakes	Bulgar Chili Bean Soup	Creamy Apple Cake	Linguine with Green Sauce
Day 6	Avocado Sesame Bread	Crispy Pasta Pea	Summer Yellow Smoothie	Bulgar Chili Bean Soup
Day 7	Roasted Pears with Walnuts	Coconut Potato Flower Stew	Pure Honey Basil	Hot Kimchi Bowl
Day 8	Blueberry Pancakes	Pure Green Soup	Summer Yellow Smoothie	Yummy spaghetti squash
Day 9	Blueberry Chia Oats	Super Hot Cucumber Soup	Pure Green Smoothie	Yummy spaghetti squash
Day 10	Avocado Sesame Bread	Bulgar Chili Bean Soup	Brain-Boosting Smoothie	Fried Leeks with Thyme
Day 11	Vegetable Tortilla	Lentil Green salad	Delicious Rosemary Pears	Mixed Beans Chili
Day 12	Blueberry Chia Oats	Scrambled Spinach Tempeh	Delicious Rosemary Pears	Yummy spaghetti squash

Day 13	Vegetable Tortilla	Coconut Potato Flower Stew	Yummy Melono Mint	Fried Leeks with Thyme
Day 14	Avocado Sesame Bread	Green Beans with Pine Nuts	Summer Yellow Smoothie	Linguine with Green Sauce
Day 15	Roasted Pears with Walnuts	Crispy Pasta Pea	Pure Green Smoothie	Hot Kimchi Bowl
Day 16	Vegetable Tortilla	Pure Green Soup	Delicious Rosemary Pears	Yummy spaghetti squashYummy spaghetti squash
Day 17	Blueberry Pancakes	Peanut Pumpkin Soup	Pure Honey Basil	Yummy spaghetti squash
Day 18	Blueberry Chia Oats	Coconut Potato Flower Stew	Brain-Boosting Smoothie	Mixed Beans Chili
Day 19	Avocado Sesame Bread	Lentil Green salad	Yummy Melono Mint	Hot Kimchi Bowl
Day 20	Blueberry Chia Oats	Pure Green Soup	Delicious Rosemary Pears	Yummy spaghetti squash
Day 21	Blueberry Pancakes	Lentil Green salad	Creamy Apple Cake	Linguine with Green Sauce

CHAPTER7:
Plant Based Diet Recipes

Breakfast Recipes

Recipe 1: Avocado Sesame Bread

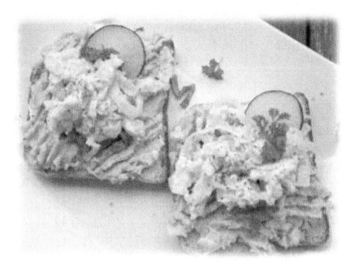

Ingredients
- Sesame bread 1
- Sliced large avocado ½
- Fresh lemon juice 2 tsp.
- Salt and black pepper to taste
- Radish slices 2
- Tomato slices 2

Preparation Method
1. At first, splits and toast the sesame bread.
2. In a small bowl, add avocado with the lemon juice, salt and pepper then divide evenly, spread the bread with the avocado mixture and top with the radishes, tomato to enjoy an extra yummy taste.

Nutritional Information

- Preparation Time: 5minutes
- Total servings: 1
- Calories: 391(per serving)
- Fat:15g
- Protein: 11g
- Carbs: 44g

Recipe 2: Blueberry Pancakes

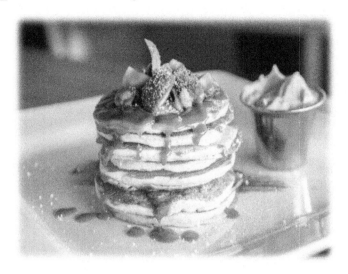

Ingredients

- Ground linseed 1 tbsp.
- Vegetable butter 1 tbsp.
- Soy milk ½ cup
- Apple cider 1 tsp.
- Millet flour 1 cup
- Baking powder 1 tsp.
- Sea salt to taste
- Blueberries 2 oz.
- Extra virgin oil 1 tsp.
- Cold water 2 tbsp.

Extra flavor

- Maple syrup

Preparation Method

1. At first, whisk linseed in cold water, then set aside to thicken. Meanwhile, melt the butter in a small pan over a medium heat then let it cool.

2. Now, combine soy milk, apple cider and add to the melted butter then whisk in the linseed mixture.
3. Combine the flour, baking powder, salt, gradually pour in the wet mixture, with constant stirring until it combined. Fold the blueberries, and set aside.
4. Preheat oven at low temperature then heats a splash of virgin oil in a large frying pan over a medium heat. Add a scoop of dough in the pan then add more scoop of dough, ensuring that it is nicely round shape.
5. Deeply cook each side for 2 minutes and place in the oven to keep warm while making remaining pancakes.
6. Serve with soy yogurt, maple syrup, and extra blueberries if desired to enjoy the taste.

Nutritional Information

- Preparation Time: 20 minutes
- Total servings: 4
- Calories: 178 (per serving)
- Fat: 6.9g
- Protein: 4.8g
- Carbs: 25.3g

Recipe 3: Roasted Pears with Walnuts

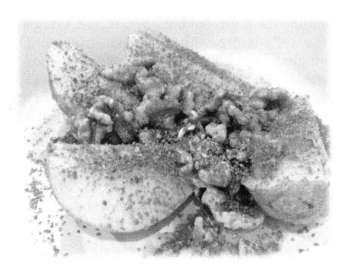

Ingredients

- Pears 5
- Cinnamon powder 1 tsp.
- Cumin seeds 1 tsp.
- Walnut halves 2 oz. (crushed)
- Pine nuts 4 tsp.

Optional

- Ginger stem 1 tbsp.

Preparation Method

1. At first, preheat your oven to 180°C. Boil (2 minutes) and cut the pears then place on oven-proof form then sprinkle cinnamon and place in oven for 20 minutes or until they brown only at the edges, let cool down.
2. Now, toast the walnuts and pine nuts in the oven for 5 minutes, save few roasted pine nuts for serving.
3. Now blend pears, ginger stem, roasted nuts until quite smooth then divide the pear mixture into 4 parts.

4. Finally, decorate with chopped toasted pine nuts, cumin seeds and serve immediately to enjoy delicious taste.

Nutritional Information

- Preparation Time: 50 minutes
- Total servings: 4
- Calories: 162 (per serving)
- Fat: 5.4g
- Protein: 1.9g
- Carbs: 23.9g

Recipe 4: Vegetable Tortilla

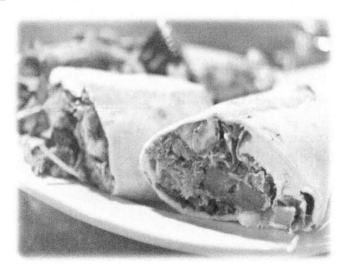

Ingredients

- Fennel slices 2
- Red peppers slices 2
- Parsley leaves 2 tbsp.
- Kalamata olives 2 tbsp.
- Fresh lemon juice 1 tbsp.
- Olive oil 2 tsp.
- Salt and black pepper to taste
- 1 tortilla, halved
- Hummus ¼ cup

Preparation Method

1. In a medium bowl, combine the fennel, peppers, parsley, olives, lemon juice, olive oil, salt, and pepper.
2. Shape sandwiches with tortilla, hummus, vegetables and enjoy the taste.

Nutritional Information

- Preparation Time: 10 minutes
- Total servings: 1
- Calories: 338 (per serving)

- Fat: 8.2g
- Protein: 12g
- Carbs: 35g

Recipe 5: Blueberry Chia Oats

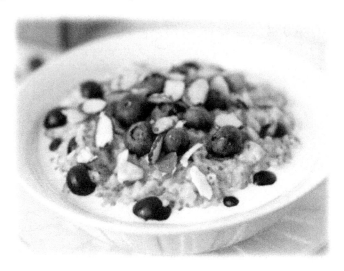

Ingredients

- Vegetable butter 1 tsp.
- Oats 1 cup
- Water 3 cups
- Coconut sugar 1 oz.
- Lemon zest 1 tbsp.
- Fresh blueberries 150g
- Chia seeds ¼ cup
- Almond flakes 2 tbsp.

Preparation Method

1. At first, place your pot on medium heat and add vegetable butter. When butter is melted, add oats and toast, regularly stir until it smells nutty (approx. 2 minutes).
2. Add water, sugar, zest, and cook for 10 minutes then stir oats, blueberries, and chia seeds.
3. Cover and let sit 5 minutes until oats comes to desired thickness. Finally, top with additional blueberries, raw honey, almonds flakes, and enjoy the taste.

Nutritional Information

- Preparation Time: 20 minutes
- Total Servings: 2
- Calories: 210
- Fat: 5g
- Protein: 8.1g
- Carbohydrates: 30.3g

Lunch Recipes

Recipe 6: Lentil Green salad

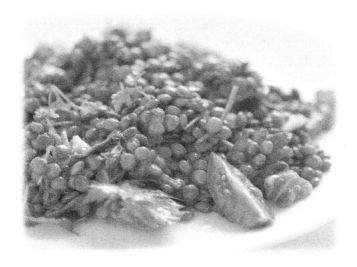

Ingredients

- Lentils 7 oz.
- Spring onions 1 bunch
- Cherry tomatoes 4 oz.
- Fresh flat parsley 1 bunch
- Fresh mint 1 bunch
- Olive oil 2 tbsp.
- Lemon juice 2 tbsp.
- Lemon zest 1 tsp.
- Himalaya sea salt ½ tsp.
- Black pepper to taste

Preparation Method

1. At first, rinse the lentils then boil in the salt water until it is tender then drain and allow cooling.
2. Meanwhile, trim and finely chop the spring onions, halve the tomatoes, then herb leaves.
3. Finally, mix the chilled lentils with spring onions, tomatoes, herbs, vegetable oil, lemon juice, zest, season

with salt and black pepper and then serve to enjoy mouthwatering herb salad taste.

Nutritional Information

- Preparation Time: 30 minutes
- Total servings: 4
- Calories: 288 (per serving)
- Fat: 14.5g
- Protein: 13.7g
- Carbs: 27.7g

Recipe 7: Green Beans with Pine Nuts

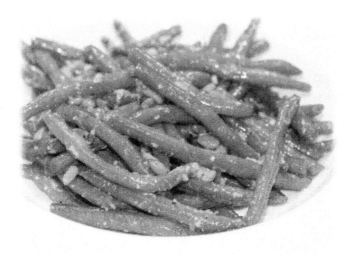

Ingredients
- Green beans 1.5 lb.
- Olive oil 2 tbsp.
- Garlic powder 1 tsp.
- Pine nuts 2 oz.
- Salt and pepper to taste

Preparation Method
1. At first, place a large pot of salt water to boil over medium heat then add the green beans and cook until tender, about 4 minutes.
2. Now, heat the vegetable oil in a large skillet over medium heat then add the garlic, pine nuts and cook for 3 minutes.
3. When green beans are cooked, drain and place on the pan. Add salt, pepper and toss to coat.
4. Finally, transfer coated green beans to a bowl and enjoys the taste.

Nutritional Information
- Preparation Time: 15 minutes
- Total servings: 6

- Calories: 140 (per serving)
- Fat: 4g
- Protein: 5.1g
- Carbs: 9.5g

Recipe 8: Scrambled Spinach Tempeh

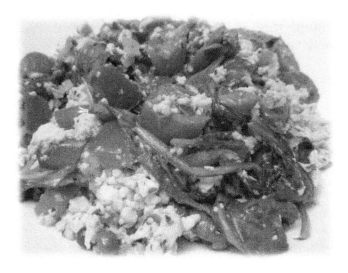

Ingredients
- Tempeh 0.9 lb.
- Ground turmeric ½ tsp.
- Salt and pepper to taste
- Cayenne pepper ½ tsp.
- Extra virgin oil 2 tbsp.
- Sliced scallions 3
- Chopped spinach 5 oz.
- Fresh lemon juice 2 tsp.
- Grape tomatoes 3 oz.
- Basil 1 tbsp.

Preparation Method
1. In a medium bowl, mix tofu, black pepper, salt, cayenne and set aside.
2. Place a pan over medium heat and add oil, scallion and cook until it looks soft then add tofu mixture and stir well until tofu turns to brown color, approximately 5 minutes.
3. Now, add spinach, lemon juice, tomatoes and salt and cook for 1 minute. Turn off the heat and add chopped basil over it to enjoy the delicious taste.

Nutritional Information

- Preparation Time: 25 minutes
- Total servings: 2
- Calories: 320 (per serving)
- Fat: 11g
- Protein: 21g
- Carbs: 15g

Recipe 9: Coconut Potato Flowerdew

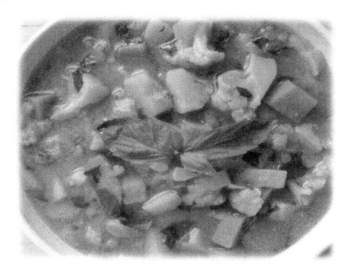

Ingredients

- Onions 2 oz.
- Garlic powder 1 tsp.
- Ginger powder 1 tsp.
- Ghee 2 tsp.
- Potatoes½ lb.
- Cauliflower 5 oz.
- Coconut milk 1 cup
- Coriander 1 tbsp.
- Cumin powder 1 tsp.
- Green chili 1 tsp.
- Turmeric 1 tsp.
- Carrot 2 oz.
- Tomatoes 1 oz.
- Water ½ cup
- Salt and fresh pepper to taste

Preparation Method

1. Heat in a large skillet pan; add ghee and onions on medium heat. Cook about 10 minutes. Add garlic and ginger, cook for another 2 minutes.

2. Add potatoes, cauliflower to the pan and brown. Season with salt, pepper, cumin, coriander, green chili, turmeric and mix well.
3. Add coconut milk, carrot, tomato, and water. Reduce heat to simmer about 30 minutes or until desired taste comes.

Nutritional Information

- Preparation Time: 35 minutes
- Total servings: 4
- Calories: 280.3 (per serving)
- Fat: 9g
- Protein: 17.1g
- Carbs: 32.1g

Recipe 10: Crispy Pasta Pea

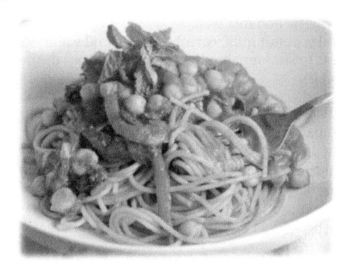

Ingredients

- Pasta ¾ lb.
- Chickpeas 15 oz.
- Capers ¼ cup
- Vegetable oil 1 tbsp.
- Garlic cloves 2
- Ginger ½ tsp.
- Ground coriander ½ tsp.
- Salt and black pepper to taste
- Fresh cilantro leaves ¼ cup
- Fresh lemon juice 2 tbsp.

Preparation Method

1. At first, preheat your oven to 400°F. Cook the spaghetti according to the given instructions on packet then drain and put in the pot.
2. Meanwhile, mix chickpeas, capers, vegetable oil, garlic, ginger, coriander, salt, pepper then place in oven and roast for 15 minutes or until it becomes crispy.
3. Finally, add roasted chickpeas mixture, lemon juice, and chopped cilantro to the pasta and toss to combine. If desired, add little vinegar and enjoy the taste.

Nutritional Information

- Preparation Time: 35minutes
- Total servings: 4
- Calories: 441 (per serving)
- Fat: 10g
- Protein: 16g
- Carbs:42g

Dinner Recipes

Recipe 11: Mixed Beans Chili

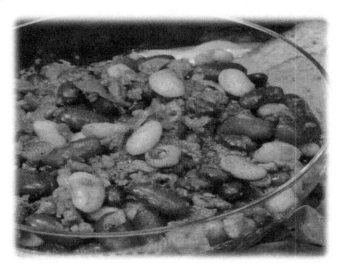

Ingredients
- Vegetable oil 1 tbsp.
- Onions ¼ cup
- Carrots ¼ cup (diced)
- Tomatoes 14 oz. (diced)
- Himalaya salt 1/2 tsp.
- Black pepper to taste
- Chickpeas 15 oz.
- White beans 15 oz.
- Kidney beans 15 oz.
- Garlic powder 2 tsp.
- Fresh parsley 1 cup
- Water 2 cups

Preparation Method
1. At first, heat Vegetable oil in a large pot over medium heat and add onions, carrots and cook until tender, about 5 minutes.

2. Now, add tomatoes, water, salt, pepper and bring to a boil. After 5 minutes, add the chickpeas, white beans, kidney beans and cook until heated, about 5 minutes.
3. In a small bowl, mix garlic, parsley, vegetable oil, and salt. Divide cooked beans into the individual bowls and top with the yogurt. Serve with the bread to enjoy an extra taste.

Nutritional Information

- Preparation Time: 20 minutes
- Total servings: 4
- Calories: 308 (per serving)
- Fat: 6g
- Protein: 12g
- Carbs: 43g

Recipe 12: Fried Leeks with Thyme

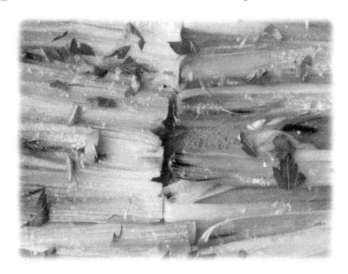

Ingredients

- Leeks 20
- Vegetable oil 2 tbsp.
- Red wine vinegar 2 tbsp.
- Fresh thyme leaves 1 tsp.
- Garlic cloves 2

Preparation Method

1. At first, preheat your oven to 400°F. Remember 5 leeks per person, depending on the size you are using.
2. Now, quickly cut both ends and peel back the first or second layer of leek leaves, then boil in a pan with salt water for 2 minutes.
3. Drain and mix with Vegetable oil, red wine, chopped thyme leaves and garlic. Evenly spread the leeks in a layer on a baking tray and cook for about 10 minutes in the oven until it caramelizes.

Nutritional Information

- Preparation Time: 20 minutes
- Total servings: 4
- Calories: 76 (per serving)

- Fat: 2g
- Protein: 3g
- Carbs: 5.2g

Recipe 13: Yummy spaghetti squash

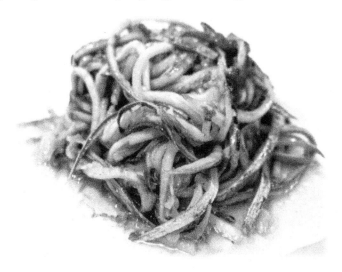

Ingredients

- Tempeh 0.7 lb.
- Tamari 1 tbsp.
- Soy sauce 1 oz.
- Garlic cloves 2
- Spaghetti squash2 lb.
- Olive oil 1 tbsp.
- Noodle sauce 1 lb.
- Broccoli flowers 2 cups
- Spinach 2 oz.

Preparation Method

1. At first, preheat your oven to 375°F. In a medium bowl, mix tempeh, tamari, garlic and set aside for 30 minutes.
2. Cook squash halves for 30 minutes and set aside. Now add oil in a large pan over medium heat and fry tempeh mixture for 8 minutes, add remaining ingredients such as sauce, broccoli, spinach and boil for 5 minutes.
3. Finally, add to serving plate and enjoy with your favorite spices to get an extra taste.

Nutritional Information

- Preparation Time: 90 minutes
- Total servings: 4
- Calories: 330 (per serving)
- Fat: 10g
- Protein: 22g
- Carbs: 27g

Recipe 14: Hot Kimchi Bowl

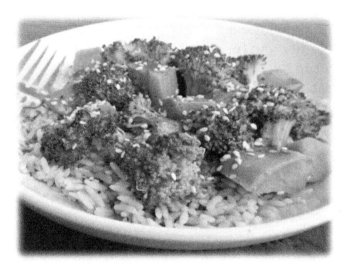

Ingredients

- Sweet potatoes 2 (cubed & roasted)
- Brown rice 2 (cooked)
- Heads broccoli 2 (roasted)
- Lentils 28 oz. (cooked)
- Kimchi 2 cups
- Fennel seeds 1 tsp.
- Black sesame seeds 1 tsp.
- Chili flakes 1 tsp.

Sauce:

- Yellow miso 1 tbsp.
- Tahini 2 tbsp.
- Lemon juice 3 tbsp.
- Water 3 tbsp.
- Cayenne pepper 1 tsp.

Preparation Method

1. At first, combine sauce ingredients in a small bowl, then stir until smooth and creamy (add more water to thin if desired).
2. Now, place the sweet potatoes, rice, broccoli, lentils, and kimchi in bowls then top with sauce, fennel seeds, black sesame seeds and chili flakes.

Nutritional Information

- Preparation Time: 5 minutes
- Total servings: 4
- Calories: 291 (per serving)
- Fat: 5.8g
- Protein: 6.6g
- Carbs: 42.2g

Recipe 15: Linguine with Green Sauce

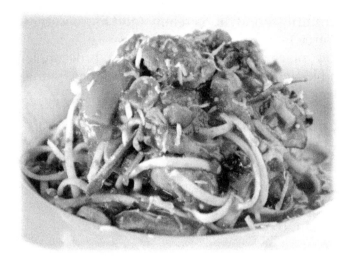

Ingredients
- Olive oil 1 tbsp.
- Garlic cloves 2
- Red pepper flakes ¼ tsp.
- Marinara/tomato sauce 25 oz.
- Spanish 1 oz.
- Green olives 4
- Capers 2 oz.
- Parsley ½ cup
- Lemons zest ½ tsp.
- Linguine (noodles) 1 lb.

Preparation Method
1. At first, heat the olive oil over medium heat then add garlic, red pepper to skillet until fragrant, approximately 2 minutes.
2. Now, add the marinara/tomato sauce, spinach, olives, capers, parsley, lemons zest and cook on simmer for 15 minutes.
3. Meanwhile, cook the linguine according to the instructions given on packet and pour the sauce over linguine and enjoy the taste.

Nutritional Information

- Preparation Time: 20 minutes
- Total servings: 4
- Calories: 346 (per serving)
- Fat: 7g
- Protein: 12g
- Carbs: 37g

Soup Recipes

Recipe 16: Pure Green Soup

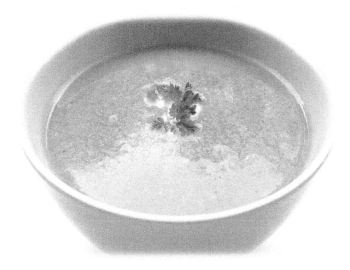

Ingredients
- Onions ½ cup
- Celery sticks 2
- Leek 1
- Garlic cloves 2
- Olive oil as needed
- Potatoes 3
- Zucchinis 2
- Sea salt to taste
- Fresh black pepper to taste
- Fresh vegetables broth 4 cups
- Fresh peas 4 oz.
- Fresh spinach ½ lb.
- Fresh mint to taste

Preparation Method
1. At first, place a large saucepan over medium heat and add chopped onions, celery, leeks, garlic, olive oil and vegetable broth, close the lid and cook for 15 minutes.

2. Meanwhile, cut potatoes, zucchinis in 2 cm chunks and put in a saucepan. Now, add a pinch of salt and pepper for better taste and continue to cook for another 15 minutes or until the potato is boiled properly.
3. Now, add the peas and the spinach and cook for 5 more minutes. Using a blender, blend the mixture until smooth. Check once the taste and add salt and pepper, if desired.
4. Finally, add chopped mint leaves, discard the stalks and enjoy delicious soup.

Nutritional Information

- Preparation Time: 40 minutes
- Total servings: 8
- Calories: 125 (per serving)
- Fat: 4.5g
- Protein: 5.5g
- Carbs: 13.7g

Recipe 17: Peanut Pumpkin Soup

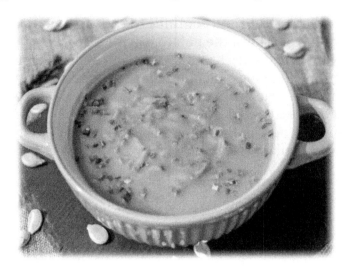

Ingredients

- Avocado oil 2 tbsp.
- Onions 1 cups
- Fresh ginger 1 tbsp.
- Green chili 1
- Garlic cloves 3
- Himalaya salt 2 tsp.
- Cumin powder 1 tsp.
- Vegetable broth 4 cups
- Tomato puree 2 cups
- Acorn pumpkin 1 (small chunks)
- Black peas 16 oz.
- Coriander leaves 1 tsp.

Preparation Method

1. At first, heat the oil in a pan over medium heat then add the onions and cook for 5 minutes then add the ginger, chili, garlic, salt, cumin and cook for 2 more minutes.
2. Now, add the broth, tomato puree, acorn pumpkin and cook until the pumpkin is tender about 30 minutes.

3. Finally, add the black peas and cook for 5 minutes. Using a blender, blend mixture into a smooth puree.
4. Before serving sprinkle with chopped coriander leaves for extra taste.

Nutritional Information

- Preparation Time: 50 minutes
- Total servings: 4
- Calories: 366 (per serving)
- Fat: 8g
- Protein: 18g
- Carbs: 38g

Recipe 18: Melono Yummy Soup

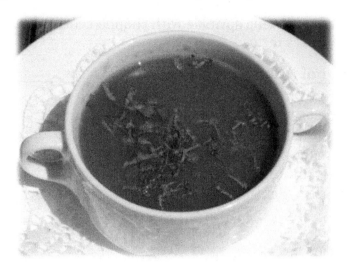

Ingredients

- Fresh tomatoes 2 cups
- Fresh watermelon 2 cups
- Fresh peppers 2
- Red onions ¼ cup
- Lime juice 1 tbsp.
- Salt ½ tsp.
- Fresh black pepper ½ tsp.
- Fresh basil leaves ¼ cup

Preparation Method

1. At first, place tomatoes, watermelon, pepper, onions in a pan and blend until thoroughly pureed.
2. Add the remaining ingredients except for basil, and blend to combine. Cook for 60 minutes in simmer and serve with basil leaves for yummy taste.

Nutritional Information

- Preparation Time: 60 minutes
- Total servings: 4
- Calories: 110 (per serving)
- Fat: 1.2g

- Protein: 3g
- Carbs: 15g

Recipe 19: Super Hot Cucumber Soup

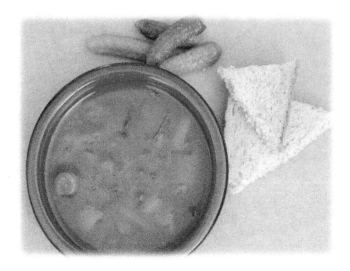

Ingredients

- Tomatoes 2
- Cucumber 1
- Onion ½ cup
- Green pepper ½ piece
- Garlic clove 1
- Wine vinegar 1 tbsp.
- Red pepper sauce 2 tsp.
- Pink salt ¼ tsp.
- Spicy hot vegetable stock 2 cups

Preparation Method

1. At first, in a large bowl mix all ingredients and cook for 30 minutes over medium heat.
2. Let it cool for 10 minutes and serve to enjoy spicy soup taste.

Nutritional Information

- Preparation Time: 40 minutes
- Total servings: 2
- Calories: 40 (per serving)

- Fat: 0.5g
- Protein: 2.8g
- Carbs: 8g

Recipe 20: Bulgar Chili Bean Soup

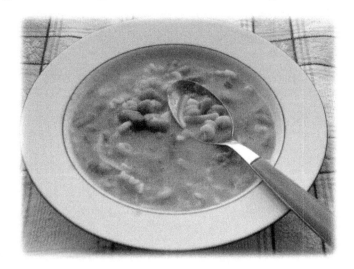

Ingredients

- Bulgur ½ cup
- Water 3 cup
- Olive oil 2 tbsp.
- Onions ½ cup
- Green peppers 1 (chopped)
- Garlic cloves 2
- Caraway powder 1 tsp.
- Chili powder 1 tsp.
- Salt and black pepper to taste
- Tomatoes 14 oz. (diced)
- White beans 15 oz.
- Fresh lemon juice 1 tbsp.
- Shallots 2 (chopped)
- Jalapeno 1(chopped)

Preparation Method

1. At first, bring 1 cup of water to boil then add bulgur and cook until all the water is absorbed and the bulgur is tender approximately 12 to 15 minutes.

2. Meantime, heat olive oil in a pot over medium heat and add onions, pepper and cook until tender, approximately 8 minutes.
3. Now, add garlic, green pepper, chili powder, salt, pepper and cook until fragrant. Add tomatoes and 2 cups of water. Bring to a boil and add beans until slightly thickened, approximately 10 minutes.
4. Add lemon juice, shallots, jalapeno, remaining olive oil, salt, and pepper in the bulgur.

Nutritional Information

- Preparation Time: 40 minutes
- Total servings: 4
- Calories: 269 (per serving)
- Fat: 6g
- Protein: 11g
- Carbs: 39g

Dessert Recipes

Recipe 21: Chocolate Brownies

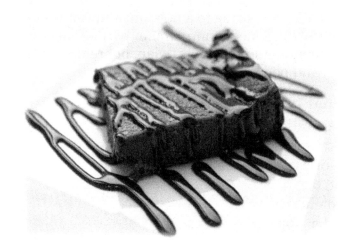

Ingredients

- Flaxseed powder 6 tbsp.
- Water 9 tbsp.
- Kidney beans 14 oz. (make paste)
- Brown sugar 200g
- Cocoa powder 2 oz.
- Ground almonds 2 oz.
- Olive oil 1 tbsp.
- Sunflower oil 1 tbsp.
- Baking powder 1 tsp.
- Vanillas extract 1 tsp.
- Vegan dark chocolate 3.5 oz.

For coconut cream:

- Coconut Cream 200ml
- Icing sugar 3 tbsp.
- Vanillas extract ½ tsp.

Preparation Method

1. At first, before you make brownies, put your coconut cream in the refrigerator for 24 hours. Preheat the oven to 180°C, apply oil to brownie tins or plate and set aside.
2. In a small bowl, mix flaxseed powder with water, stir well and allow thickening on one side.
3. Add kidney beans paste, sunflower oil, sugar, cocoa, ground almonds, baking soda, vanillas extract to the flaxseed mixture and mix until you get a shiny dough.
4. Now, cut the dark chocolate into small pieces then add to mixture. Spoon the dough into the prepared brownie tin and bake for 60 minutes.
5. In a small bowl, beat the chilled coconut cream, icing sugar, and vanilla extract until a thick and creamy paste.
6. Cut the brownie into squares and serve with the coconut cream to enjoy a yummy taste.

Nutritional Information

- Preparation Time: 70 minutes
- Total servings: 9
- Calories: 340 (per serving)
- Fat: 7g
- Protein: 11g
- Carbs: 42g

Recipe 22: Creamy Apple Cake

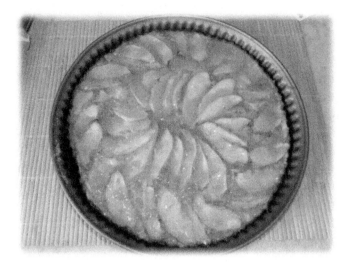

Ingredients

- Vegetable butter 1 oz.
- Apples 3
- Sugar 7 oz.
- Buckwheat flour1 cup
- Baking powder 1 tsp.
- Allspice 1 tsp.
- Sunflower oil as needed
- Vinegar 1 tsp.
- Lemon zest 1
- Walnuts 85g
- Water 180ml

Preparation Method

1. At first, preheat your oven to 180°C and grease cake mold with vegetable butter.
2. Slice the 2 apples and keep aside. Mix sugar and melted butter in a pan, then add to cake mold and top with the apple slices in a single layer.
3. Now, mix buckwheat flour, sugar, baking soda and mixed spices in a bowl. In another bowl, combine the

oil, water, vinegar, grated 1 apple and lemon zest. Mix the dry ingredients with the wet, quick, but thorough.

4. Chop the walnuts roughly then pour over the apple layer in the cake mold and bake for 30 minutes.
5. Allow the cake to cool for 5 minutes and enjoy the taste.

Nutritional Information

- Preparation Time: 45 minutes
- Total servings: 9
- Calories: 340 (per serving)
- Fat: 9.9g
- Protein: 6.8g
- Carbs: 39.6g

Recipe 23: Delicious Rosemary Pears

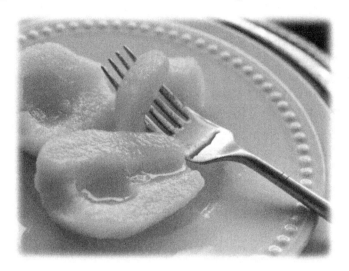

Ingredients

- Fresh pears 3
- Fresh orange juice ¼ cup
- Fresh rosemary 1 tbsp.
- Palm sugar ¼ cup

Preparation Method

1. At first, cut the pears then spread the wedges on dessert plates. Pour the orange juice over pear wedges.
2. Combine the rosemary, sugar and sprinkle over the pears to enjoy the delicious taste.

Nutritional Information

- Preparation Time: 10 minutes
- Total servings: 4
- Calories: 177 (per serving)
- Fat: 0.3g
- Protein: 1g
- Carbs: 26g

Recipe 24: Yummy Melono Mint

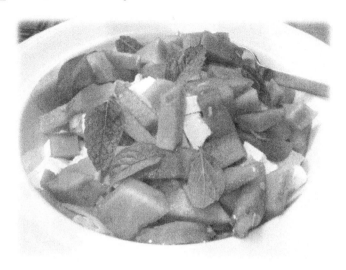

Ingredients

- Watermelon 1 lb.
- Fresh mint ½ bunch
- Lime juice 1 tbsp.
- Lime zest 1 tbsp.
- Coconut sugar ¾ cup

Preparation Method

1. At first, cut the watermelon into 2-inch thick rounds and cut each in 4 wedges.
2. In a medium bowl, add chopped mint leaves, lime zest, sugar and mix well.
3. Finally, place the watermelon on a serving plate; squeeze the lime juice over the wedges, sprinkle mint lime sugar over it and enjoy the taste.

Nutritional Information

- Preparation Time: 10 minutes
- Total servings: 6
- Calories: 148 (per serving)

- Fat: 0.2g
- Protein: 2g
- Carbs: 29g

Recipe 25: Pure Honey Basil

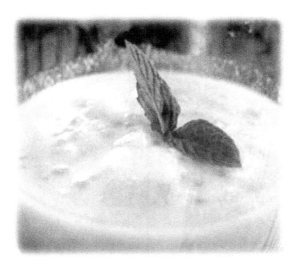

Ingredients

- Honey melon 5 lb.
- Sparkling wine 1 cup
- Fresh basil leaves ¼ cup

Preparation Method

1. At first, using a soup spoon, cut the half of a honey melon into small pieces and divide it under a bowl.
2. Now, pour 1 cup of sparkling wine over the honey melon, sprinkle fresh basil leaves and enjoy the yummy taste.

Nutritional Information

- Preparation Time: 5 minutes
- Total servings: 4
- Calories: 97 (per serving)
- Fat: 0.1g
- Protein: 1g
- Carbs: 14g

Smoothies Recipes

Recipe 26: Pure Green Smoothie

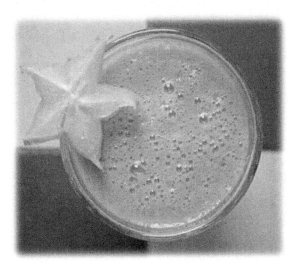

Ingredients
- Banana 1
- Fresh spinach 200g
- Fresh apple juice 250ml
- Lime juice 2 tbsp.

Preparation Method
1. At first, peel the banana and cut into small slices then blend banana and spinach in a blender.
2. Now, add that blended puree in the apple juice then add lime juice and mix well.
3. If desired, before serving add little coconut cream over it and enjoy the delicious smoothie.

Nutritional Information
- Preparation Time: 5minutes
- Total servings: 2
- Calories: 176 (per serving)
- Fat: 1.2g
- Protein: 4g
- Carbs: 30.1g

Recipe 27: Strawberry Milk Smoothie

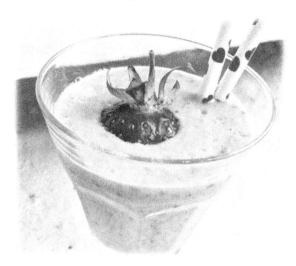

Ingredients

- Frozen strawberries 150g
- Coconut milk 240ml
- Almond butter 30g
- Stevia 10 drops

Preparation Method

1. Add all the ingredients to the blender and blend until it becomes smooth.
2. Pour into the glass and enjoy the delicious taste.

Nutritional Information

- Preparation Time: 10 minutes
- Total servings: 2
- Calories: 52 (per serving)
- Fat: 2.3g
- Protein: 0.3g
- Carbs: 10.6g

Recipe 28: Beet Carrot Smoothie

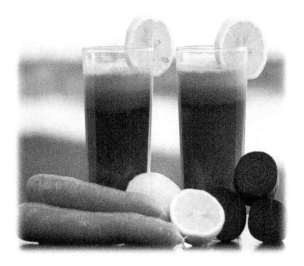

Ingredients

- Carrot 2 oz.
- Beets 2 oz.
- Fresh mint 1 oz.
- Lemon juice 2 tbsp.
- Fresh ginger 1 tbsp.
- Star anise 1

Preparation Method

1. Add all the ingredients to the blender and blend until it becomes smooth.
2. Pour into serving glass and enjoy the taste.

Nutritional Information

- Preparation Time: 10 minutes
- Servings per Recipe: 1
- Calories: 108
- Fat: 1g
- Protein: 3.3g
- Carbs: 16g

Recipe 29: Brain-Boosting Smoothie

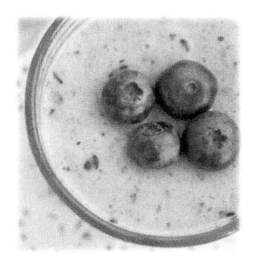

Ingredients
- Walnuts 6
- Banana 1
- Blueberries 3 oz.
- Almond milk 1 ½ cup
- Mango 2 oz.

Preparation Method
1. Add all the ingredients to the blender and blend until it becomes smooth.
2. Pour into serving glass and enjoy the taste.

Nutritional Information
- Preparation Time: 10 minutes
- Servings per Recipe: 1
- Calories: 311
- Fat: 4.9g
- Protein: 9.1g
- Carbs: 18g

Recipe 30: Summer Yellow Smoothie

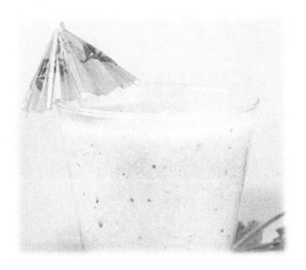

Ingredients

- Yellow summer squash 5 oz.
- Asparagus 5 oz.
- Celery 2.5 oz.
- Mint 2 oz.
- Garlic 4 tsp.

Preparation Method

1. Add all the ingredients to the blender and blend until it becomes smooth.
2. Pour into serving glass and enjoy the taste.

Nutritional Information

- Preparation Time: 5 minutes
- Servings per Recipe: 2
- Calories: 167 (per serving)
- Fat: 2.2g
- Protein: 3.1g
- Carbs: 19g

CONCLUSION

The information provided in this book will help you in the right way toward your successful dream to reduce weight and maintain a lean body, good health throughout your life. Before you start each day, remember and remind yourself about incredible benefits you achieve while doing this diet and tell yourself that you can do this for improving your health and vitality. Don't forget to take measurements and photos before you start your diet; this is the best way to monitor your progress and remember this is not just for weight loss, this is for achieving better health throughout your life. Once again thank you for choosing this book, and I hope you will achieve your dream weight and health!

ABOUT THE AUTHOR

Hello! I'm Rebecca Bellis, passionate follower of a Plant based diet. I have been espousing plant based diet since 20 years old. A plant based diet is not a diet; it is a pure green lifestyle. While following this way of life, you are going to improve your health and beauty. I sincerely recommend you to follow a plant based diet and explore benefits yourself!

Made in the USA
Columbia, SC
03 May 2018